LIVING WITH LIFE-THREATENING FOOD ALLERGIES

A TEENAGER'S GUIDE TO DOING IT WELL

Elisa Stavola

edited by James Holbrooks

ACKNOWLEDGEMENTS

I'd like to thank everyone who's helped me in the compilation of this book. I'm thrilled to have gotten the chance to share my advice about living with food allergies with others. I believe anyone, whether they have food allergies or not, can benefit from this book. I'd especially like to thank Food Allergy Research and Education (FARE) and Food Allergy and Anaphylaxis Connection Team (FAACT) for providing me with the background material used in the reference section of this book.

ABOUT THE AUTHOR

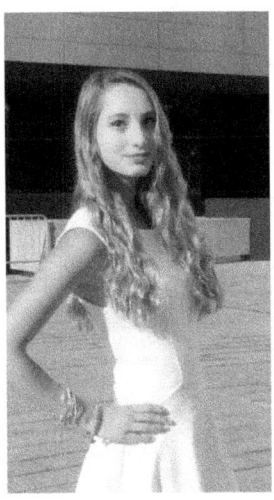

Elisa Stavola is a seventeen-year-old high school student who has suffered from food allergies her entire life.

She's very active in her high school, where she is editor of the foreign language literary magazine and captain of the varsity field hockey team. She's a member of numerous national honor societies and is involved in several volunteering programs. She was also nominated to participate in HOBY, the Hugh O'Brian Youth Leadership Foundation, an internationally recognized organization.

In the fall of 2014, Elisa received the President's Volunteer Service Award from President Barack Obama for her outstanding contribution of both time and effort in community service.

She is a teen advisor on both the Teen Advisory Group for FARE and the Teen Advisory Council for FAACT. These groups help educate the public about food allergies and advise teens on how to manage their condition.

CONTENTS

PART ONE: ME

When I was one year old my parents found out the hard way that I had food allergies. The first time I had a reaction my family was on vacation in Puerto Rico. My mom had given me a small piece of smoked turkey, and in no time hives had broken out all over my body and my eyes had swelled shut. Knowing something was very wrong, my mom called the hotel doctor. He administered Benadryl and informed her I was having an allergic reaction. When we got back home she called her cousin, Dr. Neal LeLeiko, a renowned pediatric gastroenterologist. It was *he* who referred us to a colleague of his at Mount Sinai Hospital in New York.

This colleague, Dr. Scott Sicherer, has remained my allergist to this day. Dr. Sicherer received his MD from Johns Hopkins University, his Residency of Pediatrics from Mount Sinai Hospital and his Fellowship of Allergy and Immunology from Johns Hopkins Hospital. He is on both the American Board of Pediatrics and the American Board of Allergy and Immunology. He is both a clinician and a clinical researcher for the Jaffe Food Allergy Institute at Mount Sinai, and in 2009 he was honored as a Best Doctor by New York Magazine.

The very plain and simple truth about growing up with food allergies is that it's difficult. In all honesty, I've often considered it a curse. I remember how it was in grade school, when I'd have to bring my own lunch and sit at a separate table—an "allergy table"—away from my friends. It was much the same at camp, where I'd have to eat a different ice pop than everyone else or have a special lunch made just for me.

It can be hard for any child to leave the familiar world of grade school behind. Middle school means new classes, new classmates, new everything. But for children with allergies it can be especially difficult. Suddenly a great deal of responsibility is heaped upon your small shoulders. No longer is there one teacher to carry around your EpiPen bag. No longer are you surrounded by kids you've known for years—ones that are already understanding of your condition.

When I entered middle school I began carrying a purse with me everywhere I went. In the purse I carried my *own* EpiPens, my *own* Benadryl. The front office and the nurse's office stored packs of these items, of course, but that wasn't good enough. I wanted to be independent. And what I found was that with the purse on my shoulder, a whole new world opened up for me. I wasn't alone, but for the first time in my life I was taking care of my own food allergies. I even started going out with my friends without the accompaniment of a parent. But more importantly, I was beginning to understand how to self-advocate on a higher level.

But as with all things in life, with added independence comes added responsibility—and it's certainly the case for those of us with food allergies. For me, things began to grow increasingly complicated in my teen years. Take dating, for instance. Imagine the type of research that goes into figuring out whether or not I can eat at the restaurant a date wants to take me to. Imagine the awkwardness in asking a date not to order that certain kind of snack at the movies. These are difficult situations, but it's precisely these types of issues that encouraged me to write this guide.

Teens already lead tumultuous lives. Adding the burden of life-threatening anaphylactic food allergies on top of it all can be absolutely overwhelming. But I want teens to know that it's still possible to live a relatively normal life. The information in this guide is intended to be a step in that direction.

Having lived with food allergies for sixteen years, I've discovered tricks that can make life easier for those with my condition. Through my personal journey, I've come to the conclusion that there are facts about food allergies teens simply *must* know. I feel my struggle has given me purpose, and that helping others cope with this condition will help me to *fulfill* that purpose. It is my hope that readers, whether they have food allergies or not, will find this resource guide informative and useful.

PART TWO: EDUCATION

Food allergies are on the rise in developed countries. Fifteen million Americans—one in every thirteen children—are affected. The reason for this spike is unknown, but what *is* known is that the rise is exponential.

A fifty percent increase in children with food allergies has been documented between 1997 and 2011. An allergic reaction that sends someone to the ER happens every three minutes. When added together, that equates to more than 200,000 trips a year.

Eight major allergens account for more than ninety percent of all allergic reactions. Those allergens are: peanuts, tree nuts, shellfish, soy, wheat, fish, milk and eggs. The risk of a child having a food allergy is higher for those born to a parent who has any type of "allergic disease" (asthma, eczema, food or environmental allergies).

Outgrowing food allergies is more common for some foods than for others. Peanuts, tree nuts, shellfish and fish, for example, tend not to be outgrown while egg and milk allergies tend to develop in childhood but be outgrown by sixteen years of age.

There is no cure. The only way to deal with food allergies is through the strict avoidance of triggers. Even trace amounts of an allergen, through cross-contamination, can lead to an anaphylactic reaction.

None of us exists in a bubble. Those of us with food allergies may live within special parameters, but that doesn't make us special. Like everyone else, we must navigate through the world as best we can. In the case of teenagers with food allergies, the best way to participate in the school environment is by educating those around you. The following is an explanation, with relevant references, of helpful ways to do just that.

NOTE: These documents may be updated yearly, so please check the corresponding websites for additional information.

Fill out the *Anaphylaxis Emergency Action Plan*, found on the American Academy of Allergy, Asthma and Immunology's website at www.aaaai.org. Also, fill out the *Food Allergy and Anaphylaxis Emergency Care Plan* found on FARE'S website at www.foodallergy.org. Give a copy to the school nurse and any other adult who might be traveling away from school with you (such as a teacher in charge of a field trip or a coach escorting you to an away game).

You, your parents, or the school nurse should hand out a copy of the *Teacher's Checklist for Managing Food Allergies* to each of your teachers. This can be found on FARE's website as well. Make any additions or revisions you feel are necessary in order to give your teachers a heads-up about your food allergies.

If you're taking the bus to school, fill out the *Bus Drivers and Transportation Checklist* found in the Education Resource Center at www.foodallergyawareness.org and follow its directions for educating your bus driver.

Educate your friends who eat lunch with you. It's important to make them understand the seriousness related to your anaphylactic food allergies, but you want to go about it without making them feel bad. What can you do (and not do), for example, if a friend pulls out a peanut butter and jelly sandwich right next to you?

DO

Ask your friend if they are eating a peanut butter and jelly sandwich. When they say yes, calmly tell them about your condition. Explain that you can't sit next to that particular food because the allergen, if airborne, can affect you. Then switch seats, and ask your friend to wash his or her hands after eating. Thank them afterwards to show how much you appreciate them trying to keep you safe. Your friends may even decide on their own to bring a different sandwich for lunch in the future, just so they can sit next to you.

DON'T

Don't freak out and run screaming from the lunchroom. This will only offend your friend and undermine the seriousness you're trying to convey to them about your condition. What you absolutely don't want is for your food allergies to be taken as a joke.

DON'T

Never let it go. Never ever let it go, even if you find yourself in an uncomfortable situation. You need to confront the problem. If you don't, you not only put yourself in danger, you ensure that uncomfortable situations like the one with the peanut butter and jelly sandwich will be a possibility every time you enter the lunchroom.

TIP: When making new friends, it's easier to casually bring up your food allergies in conversation than to be forced into an explanation during an uncomfortable situation.

Introduce your school to FAME (Food Allergy Management and Education). St. Louis Children's Hospital developed FAME to introduce allergy-friendly environments in schools for children suffering from food allergies. FAME "provides schools with the components of a comprehensive school-based food allergy program" and presents "resources and materials to area schools and families on creating a safe nurturing educational environment for children with food allergies." By introducing your school to the FAME manual and Tool-Kit, you can make your school a safer place for yourself and others with anaphylactic food allergies.

NOTE: For more information on managing food allergies see the Centers for Disease Control's *Voluntary Guidelines for Managing Food Allergies in Schools and Early Care and Education Programs*, along with its Frequently Asked Questions, on CDC's website at www.cdc.gov.

The EpiPen4Schools Program is offered by Mylan Specialty, the marketer and distributor of EpiPen and EpiPen Jr Auto-injectors. With this program, schools will have access to epinephrine in case of an anaphylactic reaction. Schools that qualify have three options: two 2-Paks of EpiPens with a trainer in each pack, two 2-Paks of EpiPen *Jrs* with a trainer in each pack, or one of *each* pack, trainers included.

And finally, a word on the law. It's very important that teens with food allergies acquaint themselves with the state and federal laws that may apply to them.

EXAMPLES OF CIVIL RIGHTS LEGISLATION

Section 504 of the Rehabilitation Act of 1973 prohibits programs receiving federal funding (public schools) from discriminating against individuals with disabilities. Section 504 defines individuals with disabilities as "persons with a physical or mental impairment which substantially limits one or more major life activities." Students with food allergies qualify for Section 504 protection because anaphylaxis impairs the "major life activity" of breathing.

The Americans with Disabilities Act (ADA) prohibits discrimination against people with disabilities and guarantees them equal opportunities.

The School Access to Emergency Epinephrine Act is a relatively new law, signed by President Obama in November of 2013, and "encourages states to adopt laws requiring schools to 'stock' epinephrine auto-injectors" by providing financial incentives for states to comply. This is an extremely important piece of legislation because twenty-five percent of first-time anaphylactic reactions in schools occur in students who were previously unaware they had a food allergy.

PART THREE: SAFETY

Educating your teachers and peers about your food allergies is a great first step in keeping yourself safe. Obviously, though, threats to your health don't begin and end at the schoolhouse doors. Teens with food allergies need to know how to ensure their own safety in a wide range of situations. There's simply no other choice for those who want to lead a full and rich life. In this section, we'll cover ways to safely interact in a number of different scenarios. We'll begin with school, which we've touched on already, then move on to more isolated activities.

LUNCHROOM

Always wash your hands before you eat—you never know what you may have come into contact with. Remember, even trace amounts of an allergen can cause a serious allergic reaction. Be mindful where you place your food on the table, especially if you're sitting close to someone else. Personally, since our lunchroom tables are always packed with kids, I've gotten into the habit of eating out of my lunchbox. This way, I'm not worried about dirty surfaces or flying food (lunchtime can get messy). If you insist on placing your food directly on the surface, however, packing wipes—such as Wet Ones—with which to first clean the table is advisable.

I used to be somewhat embarrassed to bring my not-so-stylish lunch bag to the cafeteria. This changed when I found Koko lunch bags, which are both stylish *and* convenient. You can find them at www.kokolunchbags.org. My lunch bag, which looked more like a purse, began to get me compliments. Suddenly I wasn't embarrassed to bring my lunch to school anymore.

For those times when you need to carry large amounts of food, I use bags by Lands' End. I've used their bags to bring dinner plates to restaurants and to holiday parties where I needed to bring my own food. You can find Lands' End products at www.landsend.com.

SPORTS

If you're on a sports team, as I am, alert your coach to your life-threatening allergies. If you're allergic to nuts, in particular, you should ask your coach to make an announcement requesting that the team not bring any nuts on the bus. This is due to the fact that a pack of nuts, when opened, can release dust into the air.

It can be very difficult to request that your teammates not bring snacks you're allergic to on the bus. A good alternative is to bring allergy-friendly snacks for everyone. This may alleviate the need for them to bring their own, potentially harmful foods. But if a teammate next to you *does* start to eat something you're allergic to, immediately tell them about your allergies and politely ask them to either save the snack for later or move to a different seat.

FIELD TRIPS

These situations can be more difficult to control, especially when you're traveling overnight. The key is preparation. Chaperones must be advised about your food allergies and prepared for an emergency. In theory, field trips should be planned with food-allergic students in mind, though this doesn't always happen. For example, a class shouldn't visit a ranch where peanuts are fed to animals if a student has a peanut allergy, and a class should avoid visiting an ice cream shop if students have a milk allergy.

If your class *was* taking a trip to said farm, and you were unaware of the peanuts, upon arriving it would be advisable to ask a chaperone if you could sit out the tour due to your serious condition. In the case of the ice cream shop, ask your friends to wash their hands when they're done eating. Another option is to carry wipes on the bus with you and have a chaperone pass them out to the other students once everyone is back on the bus. These tips should work very well for younger teens, but as you approach high school the trips become less structured and monitored. The truth is, it's impossible to control all aspects of the situations you find yourselves in, and it's best to focus on keeping yourself safe on a personal level.

Realistically, schools will rarely plan a trip around your food allergies. And again, it's best to take your safety into your own hands anyway. If staying overnight at a hotel, for example, call the hotel in advance to reserve a room with a refrigerator and microwave. Be sure to inform the trip chaperone that this is a requirement for you to be able to make your own food. Have a food bag packed with foods you'll eat over the course of the trip—foods that can be stored in the refrigerator upon arrival at the hotel. To keep the food fresh while traveling, load your bags down with ice packs. Bring enough to put a couple in your lunch box as well. The refrigerator in the hotel room will most likely have a freezer compartment where you can keep the ice packs.

TIP: When I'm on a class trip, I wake up an hour earlier than everyone else so I have time to eat my breakfast and pack my food for the day. That way I'm not rushing to finish packing in the morning while everyone else is ready to go.

CAMP

I never went to sleep away camp, but I *did* go to day camp. FARE has a detailed document explaining the responsibilities of the family, the camper, and the camp in making sure the camper stays safe. Here is a list of the parts that apply to you in keeping yourself safe at camp.

Choose a camp that will ensure the safety of the camper.

Notify the camp of the camper's allergies.

Speak with the camp director, counselor, and/or the division supervisor.

Provide a recent photo of the camper along with allergy documentation (such as the Anaphylaxis Emergency Action Plan or the Food Allergy and Anaphylaxis Emergency Care Plan).
The camper should be educated about what he/she can eat, how to self-inject, the symptoms of an allergic reaction, and how to stay safe (no sharing food).

When I was younger, in those summers I went to camp, my mother would get a full list of the food provided to campers and read the ingredients of each item. She'd compile a list of the foods I could eat and give it to the head chef, who would prepare me a lunch each day. My mother always ensured he understood about cross-contamination, changing his gloves and using clean utensils and surfaces. Specific brands of bread, bagels, and cheese were used every time. I would receive a copy of this list of safe foods and so would my division leader. If the snack of the day was not on my list, I would go to the kitchen and get one that was.

There was an upside to this. Even if the snack of the day was on my list, I was still allowed to pick whichever item I wanted! All my camp friends were jealous. Hey, having food allergies occasionally has its perks. I was always very close with my division leaders, while most campers only knew them in passing. Who knows more about food labels and health information than food allergy teens? We always know what we're putting in our mouths!

GOING OUT

When you're going out with friends, preparation begins before you leave the house. It all depends upon where you're going and what you're doing. If you're going to an amusement park for the day, you'll prepare differently than if you were going to dinner and a movie. It's like choosing an outfit for a specific occasion. You "outfit" yourself according to necessity.

Say you're going to an amusement park for the whole day. You'll need to eat in order to keep your energy up and enjoy yourself. In this situation, I'd bring both a lunch box and a belly bag. In the lunch box I'd have my lunch and other snacks and in the belly bag I'd carry my epinephrine auto-injectors, my ID, and my phone. Make sure you ask your friends where they want to eat lunch so you can find a locker near the restaurant to store your lunch box in. Explain to them that you *must* be able to get back to that locker for lunch.

There are usually lockers at each ride. Store your belly bag in a locker and make sure *you're* the one holding the keys so you can get to your bag any time you need to. Another option is to have the attendant hold your bag while you're on the ride. Either way, your epinephrine should be close at hand at all times.

NOTE: When out in public, you should always wear some sort of medical alert identification (a necklace, bracelet, etc.)
If you're going out for dinner and a movie with your friends, you don't have to eat before you go. You *can* eat at the restaurant, there are just some steps you have to take to stay safe.

Choosing a restaurant. Avoid super busy establishments—the busier they are, the less special attention they can give you. Don't go for the tiny restaurants, either. These are more likely to be lax in their health regulation policies. Choose restaurants that offer simple dishes so as to reduce the possibility of cross-contamination. Avoid language barriers—you and the staff should be able to communicate effectively. Stay away from places that use allergens in many of their meals, such as Asian and raw food restaurants (if you're allergic to soy or nuts) and ice cream parlors (if you're allergic to dairy). And wherever you choose to eat, always remember to ask about the establishment's allergen policy.

Making the situation clear. It may sound funny, but you should put together a "team" at any restaurant you eat at so that everyone involved with your food preparation understands your needs. For starters, you or your parents should call the restaurant ahead of time and speak with the manager and the head chef.

Give them a list of your allergies and ask them to read off the ingredients of any foods being used to prepare your meal. Remind them to check for "may contain" or "processed in the same facility" on the boxes. Make sure the surfaces and any utensils used in the preparation of your food are clean. Finally, make sure all hands were washed and that gloves were changed before handling your food.

When ordering, ask to speak to the manager. Introduce yourself, remind him that you or your parents had called beforehand, and tell him you just want to check to make sure everything is safe. When it's time to order your meal, give the waiter an allergy card (a list of your allergens) to give to the chef. Make sure to explain about your life-threatening condition and about how there mustn't be any cross-contamination. Ask the waiter to make sure the chef uses clean surfaces, clean hands, and that gloves are used in all stages of food preparation.

TIP: If one of your friends at dinner is eating something you're allergic to, remind them politely to wash their hands once they're finished. This will remind them about your allergies without having to specifically bring it up.

NOTE: FAACT's webpage has a lot of information on dining out.

Once dinner is over, you may find yourself in the snack line at the movies. If it's just you and one other friend, you'll need to make sure your friend doesn't buy a snack you're allergic to. This may be awkward, but it beats having to sit away from your friend in the theater (it could be potentially dangerous for you to sit directly next to a food that can harm you). If you're with a *group* of friends, you can avoid the awkwardness of asking someone to choose a different snack by simply telling them that you'll have to switch seats with someone else in the theater. This might get them to rethink their snack choice. As always, make sure your friends wash their hands after the movie.

TRAVELING

Having food allergies can make traveling difficult for both you and your parents. Essentially, there are two options when traveling. One, you can bring your own food. Two, you can speak to the head chef at either the hotel or nearby restaurants before you arrive to ensure they will safely prepare your meals.

If you decide to bring your food you must prepare your meals beforehand. When carrying food on an airplane you must have an official, signed medical note from your doctor to show the TSA. Usually they need to open the bags to make sure everything is what you say it is. A good idea may be to ship nonperishable food before you leave for your trip (this is especially handy when you are traveling to a country where labeling laws are different).

If you want to make your own meals there, you must have a hotel room with a kitchen or kitchenette and you must find a food store where you can shop. Fruits and vegetables can be bought anywhere with little to no risk of reaction. Despite different labeling laws, in France an apple is still an apple and a zucchini is still a zucchini. Packaged and processed foods are different, however. Before buying them, you should research the labeling laws of the country you're visiting. If you believe buying these foods isn't worth the risk, then have the packaged and processed foods you need shipped to your location from the U.S.

Clearly, transport is very important when traveling with food. Here are some handy items:

Cooler bags. Great for keeping days' worth of food good. When I can't travel with my thermoelectric cooler (such as on a class trip) I carry a large cooler tote bag. It fits easily on my shoulder while keeping my food insulated and fresh. Visit www.keepcoolusa.com for ideas.

Rolling coolers. Perfect for air travel. These coolers can be rolled through the terminal, taken apart, and easily stored in the overhead compartment. They're insulated and keep your food fresh for hours. Igloo and California Innovations make great rolling coolers.

Thermoelectric coolers. Going on a road trip? Whether your destination is across the country or just a couple of hours away, thermoelectric coolers ensure your food stays fresh. The inside remains cold for hours, even days, without ice. Once at your destination, they can be plugged in and used as a refrigerator. There are even adapters for your car. When these coolers are plugged in, the temperature inside drops drastically. Igloo, Koolatron and Coleman make great thermoelectric coolers.

If you decide to have a chef prepare your food, you must speak to the head chef and discuss meals and the safety precautions he or she must take. This discussion will be similar to the one you have when speaking with the chef/manager at a restaurant.

When I'm only traveling for a few days, it's easier for me to just bring the food I need in my thermoelectric cooler or my cooler bags. If I'm traveling for a few weeks, I bring the first few days' worth of breakfast and then find a food store that sells the brands I can eat. These packaged cereals or brands of bread and bagels are fairly easy to find. For lunch and dinner, I or one of my parents go over each meal with the head chef personally. Thankfully, I've never had a problem while adhering to this plan. In fact, most of the chefs I've dealt with have been very kind and accommodating.

While doing research for this guide, I came across Chef Keith Norman of the South Point Hotel in Las Vegas. I remembered some of my food allergy friends talking about how amazing he was in dealing with their food allergies. He dedicates himself and his kitchen staff to accommodating people with anaphylactic food allergies.

DATING

Dating is one of the most complicated ordeals in a teenager's life, and one made significantly more so when food allergies are involved. It's an awkward subject and something you might not want to discuss with your allergist. The best piece of advice I can give a food-allergic teen who is getting ready to begin dating is this: it's best if you stay in control of the situation. Only *you* know what you need to do to stay safe.

It can be really hard to tell someone you're on a date with that they can't do this or that because of your food allergies (even harder than telling your friends). But the bottom line is that if they're not willing to comply with the rules you must follow to stay safe, then they don't deserve to date you. It's as simple as that.

If you're going on a dinner date, for example, *you* pick the restaurant. Make it a place you know is safe. For me, the easiest type of restaurant to eat at on a date is a pizza parlor. That way, you can simply order a pizza and share it. Now you know the food your date is eating is allergy-friendly as well (this especially makes things easier if you're planning on a goodnight kiss!). Even if he wants a different topping than you, pizzas can be made half-and-half. This is fine, as long as the topping he chooses is not harmful to you.

If he chooses a topping you can't eat, tell him you won't be able to share a pizza with him because of your food allergies. This may be enough to get him to switch to another topping, because he might actually *want* to share a meal with you—he asked you out, after all. If he persists, tell him in a joking way that that's fine, as long as he understands he won't be getting a kiss at the end of the night. He might just think again about that topping.

NOTE: Another good thing about pizza parlors is that, since they specialize in a single dish, their pizzas are cooked in special ovens away from other foods.

If you're going to the movies, the same type of joke works for snacks. "I wouldn't buy those if you're planning on a goodnight kiss," you say with a smirk. If you prefer a more serious approach, then simply explain the situation. You could say: "I have severe food allergies and I'd really appreciate it if you picked something else." Again, if he gives you a hard time about it then he doesn't deserve you anyway. Even if you're not planning on a kiss, you won't have a very relaxing time in the theater if he's right next to you snacking on something you're allergic to for two hours.

TIP: If all the precautions involved with going on a date at a restaurant seem overwhelming, then make it easy on yourself and suggest a date that doesn't revolve around food (or, at a minimum, a picnic, so you can bring food you made yourself).

Since kissing is such a big part of dating, and since kissing someone who's just eaten foods you're allergic to is so potentially dangerous, it's worth it to take the time and go over a few things about kissing.

The big question, of course, is this: how long do you have to wait to kiss someone who's eaten something you're allergic to? There have actually been studies done on the matter.

My allergist, Dr. Scott Sicherer of Mount Sinai Hospital, conducted a study to discover how long peanut butter stayed in saliva. After a subject ate a whole peanut butter sandwich, it took four hours for the peanut butter to be completely untraceable. The study did *not* test how long chewed nuts stayed in saliva, however, only peanut butter. Rinsing the mouth, chewing gum and brushing teeth helped get rid of the allergen more quickly, but were not as effective as simply waiting four hours.

Another study showed that the most effective way to get rid of the peanut butter allergen is to wait several hours, then eat an allergen-free meal.

According to FARE, scientists have suggested that those with a peanut allergy should have their boyfriend/girlfriend wait a few hours before kissing you if they've consumed peanuts.

I'm not giving advice on how long you should wait before kissing someone who's eaten something you're allergic to. I would only do that if I knew the answer for certain, and I don't. I'm merely passing on the information I've found in my research so that teens can make that decision for themselves.

But there *are* a couple of common sense measures I feel comfortable with suggesting to any teen with food allergies who's about to start dating. One, your date should brush their teeth thoroughly and wash their hands and face before they even *think* about kissing you. And two, anyone you'd allow to touch their mouth to yours should know how to give you epinephrine, should there be an emergency.

To anyone with food allergies who's about to start dating, I would recommend the article "Dating with Allergies, a Tricky Business" by Lisa Fitterman. To anyone *dating* someone with food allergies, I would recommend reading "Do's and Don'ts of Dating Someone with a Food Allergy" by Stacy Goldberg.

PART FOUR: COLLEGE

The prospect of college can be scary for the average teen. For those of us with life-threatening food allergies it can be downright terrifying. College means you're on your own—that includes taking full responsibility for your personal safety with regard to allergens. Bottom line, the best way to ensure your safety is to find the right school.

FARE has many resources for would-be college students on a wide variety of subjects—one of which is choosing a school. Here are a few of their tips.

Make sure the dining facilities are safe by going on a tour and asking the food service director how you can verify the ingredients of each meal and exchange an unsafe entrée for one you can eat.

Some schools permit you to bring or rent a MicroFridge (a combination refrigerator and microwave), which allows you the option of preparing foods in your room. Find out if the top three schools you are considering have this option.

Research your housing options to see if you can choose a supportive friend to be your roommate or if you can live in a single room, which can help create a safe and allergen-free living environment.

FARE also provides guidance in the area of dorm life.

Orient your roommates, hallmates, and Resident Advisor by distributing your Food Allergy and Anaphylaxis Emergency Care

Plan *to all dorm staff members, and place a copy in your dorm room and your Resident Advisor's room.*

Be sure to talk to your roommates about your food allergy, how they can help keep you safe, and what to do in an emergency. Assemble emergency medical kits with medications you use to treat a reaction and a copy of your Food Allergy and Anaphylaxis Emergency Care Plan *signed by your doctor.*

Many schools have fast food outlets on campus; be sure to check out the ingredient lists.

For college students with food allergies, however, the threats won't only come from the foods themselves. On the subject of alcohol, and how it can affect reactions, FARE has this to say:

When alcohol is consumed, judgment, timing, and muscle coordination are adversely affected. Thus, people may take chances they should not, may misjudge what is occurring, and may allow food contamination to occur just by mishandling. Additionally, their ability to recognize a reaction, give themselves medications, and summon help may be affected.

Although alcohol is illegal for teens and young adults to consume until the age of twenty-one, it's a prevalent part of both high school and college life. When speaking about alcohol and food allergies, Dr. Clifton T. Furukawa, an allergist and clinical professor of pediatrics at the University of Washington School of Medicine, explained that alcohol may increase the absorption rate at which a food allergen is taken in, thereby leading to a quicker onset of symptoms. Nevertheless, it's important to note that alcohol will not hamper the effect of epinephrine. It's just as effective when you have alcohol in your system.

In addition to offering *guidance* to students, FARE has partnered with the National Foundation for Celiac Awareness, the National Association of College and University Food Services, food allergy experts, and stakeholders from colleges and universities to form CFAP, the College Food Allergy Program.

The research effort, by way of two college summits, brought together experts from over sixty-five schools and organizations to discuss the best ways to manage food allergies.

The summits had five major priorities:

To implement best practices guidelines for identifying students with food allergies and accommodating their needs via housing, dining, health, emergency and disability services.

To provide training to dining services staff via MenuTrinfo's AllerTrainU course.

To provide free training for resident assistants and other non-dining staff on food allergy 101, how to recognize a reaction, and how to talk to and educate students about food allergies.

To create a toolkit for parents and students to help them navigate the college process. The toolkit will provide useful information, such as what questions to ask when considering a college and how to advocate for yourself and manage food allergies on campus.

To initiate the creation of social groups on campuses to help mentor incoming students and to help students advocate for one another both on and off campus.

NOTE: CFAP goes into effect in the fall of 2014, initially in about five to ten schools.

On the subject of food allergies, both the school and the student have responsibilities with regard to safety. The following comments come from *College and University Guidelines for Managing Students with Food Allergies.*

STUDENT RESPONSIBILITIES

Notify the college/university of his or her allergies.

Work with the school to develop a plan that accommodates his or her needs.

Provide written medical documentation, instructions, and medications as directed by a physician, using the Food Allergy Action Plan *(available through FAAN) as a guide.*
Be proficient in the self-management of his or her food allergy including: (1) avoidance of unsafe foods (2) recognition of symptoms of allergic reactions (3) how and when to tell someone they may be having an allergy-related problem (4) knowledge of proper use of medications to treat an allergic reaction

Review policies/procedures with the school staff and his or her physician after a reaction has occurred.

Provide emergency contact information.

Carry prescribed medications at all times.

SCHOOL RESPONSIBILITIES

Be knowledgeable about and follow applicable federal laws including ADA, and any state laws that apply.

Review the health records submitted by students and physicians.

Identify a core team of, but not limited to, staff in health services, dining services, residence living, and security to work with the student and establish a food allergy management plan. Changes to the plan should be made with core team participation.

Resident Assistants (RAs) of students with food allergies should be able to identify such students and know how to access emergency assistance quickly.

Appropriate staff members, including RAs, should be taught food allergy basics, including symptoms, instructions for administering medications, and Emergency Medical Service procedures.

Designate school personnel who are properly trained to administer medications.

Review policies/prevention plan with the core team members and student after a reaction has occurred.
Follow federal/state/district laws and regulations regarding sharing medical information about the student.

PART FIVE: MORE

There's always more. More resources, more information. More items that deserve to be included. In this section of the guide, we'll look at additional sources of aid for those dealing with food allergies. And we'll begin with one of the most important subjects.

IDENTIFICATION

MedicAlert offers medical alert identification in a variety of forms. Their services cover a wide range and are available to all— seniors, adults, and children.

Children who are signed up are eligible for 24/7 emergency response. MedicAlert IDs grant emergency responders immediate access to members' health records. MedicAlert's Emergency Response Center is staffed by medically-trained personnel who then: (1) communicate vital medical information to emergency responders/medical personnel (2) transmit medical records to the responding hospital to ensure proper treatment (3) provide translation services for over 140 languages (4) contact you to relay your child's whereabouts and make certain your child is reunited with loved ones.

Other services include:

Family notification. The family is immediately notified about their child's condition and location.

Physician/provider notification. The physician is kept informed about the treatment and care the child is receiving and is kept in contact with the hospital.

EMIR (Emergency Medical Information Record). A comprehensive medical record that can be accessed by the staff and relayed to emergency responders and medical professionals.

Prescription drug discounts. Members receive a free GoodRx card, with discounts of up to eighty percent on prescriptions. Also, by visiting the GoodRx site or using the mobile app, you can compare prices between FDA-approved prescription drugs at almost any pharmacy in America.

TravelPlus. A program that (1) helps you find a doctor when you're out of the country (2) contacts your family members (3) arranges and pays up to $100,000 towards the necessary expense of evacuation to a qualified hospital in a medical emergency (4) provides 24 hour access to information services including visa, passport, and immunization requirements for your destination (5) provides coverage for pre-existing conditions. TravelPlus is active when you are traveling no more than 90 days at a time and are more than 100 miles from your primary home.

There are even more services available for adults. Additional information can be found at MedicAlert's website at www.medicalert.org.

NOTE: Allergy cards are another great way for emergency personnel to identify your condition and your medical needs. FARE created a Chef Card as part of their SafeFARE Dining Out with Food Allergies program. Visit FARE's website for an interactive Chef Card Template. I had my Chef Cards printed in many different colors and then laminated. Remember, if you're traveling in a foreign country always be sure to make Chef Cards in that country's language.

THE LAW

In recent years, states have begun to recognize the importance of setting up regulations to protect those with food allergies. Massachusetts and Rhode Island were the first to pass food allergy laws for restaurants. Some of the stipulations require that eateries must (1) have food allergy awareness posters in employee areas (2) have notices on menus asking customers to alert staff of any food allergies (3) employ "certified food production managers (i.e., restaurant managers and/or senior employees) that have received food allergy training via a video and obtained a certificate showing that they've received the training."

But it isn't only happening in restaurants. In early 2013 it was revealed that the Justice Department had reached a settlement with Lesley University after a number of students with food allergies sued over the school's failure to provide adequate dining options.

The court found that Lesley University was in violation of Title III of the Americans with Disabilities Act. Students were being made to pay for a school meal plan even though the food was not safe for them to eat. Under Title III, schools are required to meet "reasonable accommodations," but Lesley was falling short. The school was forced to put in place signs referencing specific food allergens and gluten and to designate space for food preparation for any student worried about cross-contamination with food allergens. A guideline for other schools is to follow.

And since we're back to the subject of college for a moment, a few other notes:

The Disability Service Office will work with you to create a plan for food-allergic students (though it's advisable not to contact this department until *after* you're admitted to the school).

The Housing Offices may make special accommodations for (1) living off campus (2) having a car (3) screening potential roommates (4) living alone in a dorm (5) having a refrigerator in a dorm.

Dining Services usually provide dietary specialists to help food-allergic students and allow them to meet with food service staff to discuss meals.

And just like that, we're back to...

FOOD

It's important that you read the labels of the products you buy—each and every time—because the labels are constantly subject to change. If the *size* of the product changes, for instance, the format of the label may change as well. And if there's no label at all, you simply DO NOT EAT.

NOTE: Crustacean shellfish such as crab, shrimp, and lobster are required to have labels, but mollusks such as clams and mussels have no such requirement. It's also worth noting that pet foods *often* contain allergens.

FARE has a program called Allergy Alert and Ingredient Notices that cooperates with many food manufacturers and provides information about mislabeled or recalled food as well as notifications about ingredient changes from responsible food companies. If you sign up to get these notifications, FARE will notify you by email of any changes. These alerts are only in regard to recalls involving the eight major allergens identified by the Food Allergen and Consumer Protection Act.

And speaking of FALCPA...

It should be pointed out that America's official list of major allergens (milk, egg, fish, crustacean shellfish, tree nuts, wheat, peanuts and soybeans) is less in number than that of both Canada (which includes sulfates and mustard) and the European Union (which includes sesame and lupin).

Officially, FALCPA only applies to foods regulated by the FDA, but for the sake of consistency the USDA complies as well. FALCPA applies to all items packaged by food service establishments and offered for human consumption, but doesn't apply to food items placed in a wrapper, container, or box in response to a customer's order (such as a fast food establishment). It requires that the eight major food allergens be identified in plain English on all labels. In addition, the specific allergen for tree nuts, fish, and shellfish must be stated (for example, walnut, salmon, shrimp).

There are three ways allergens can be listed:

By listing the allergen, in plain English, in the ingredients list itself (INGREDIENTS: rice, sugar, freeze-dried strawberries, wheat, milk, etc.).

By listing the allergen, in plain English, in a parenthetical immediately after the scientific ingredient term (sodium caseinate (milk), semolina (wheat), albumin (egg), etc.).

By having a separate "contains" statement immediately after or adjacent to the list of ingredients, in a font size at least as large as the ingredients list (example: "Contains milk and soy.").

Under FALCPA, there are no regulations on the use of precautionary allergen statements—sometimes termed *supplemental allergen labeling*—such as "may contain," "manufactured in a shared facility," and "processed on the same equipment."

Raw agricultural commodities (generally, fresh nuts and vegetables) are also exempt as are highly refined oils derived from one of the eight major food allergens as well as any ingredient derived from such highly refined oil.

More information on the Food Allergen and Consumer Protection Act can be found at FDA's website at www.fda.gov.

The Food Safety Modernization Act (FSMA) requires manufacturing facilities to identify and evaluate known or foreseeable hazards and develop written analyses. This covers everything from biological, chemical, physical and radiological hazards, to natural toxins, pesticides, drug residues, decomposition, parasites, allergens and unapproved food and color additives. Along with the written analysis, facilities are required to develop preventative control procedures, practices and processes to significantly minimize or prevent hazards.

And finally, for those that like to do it themselves, I've found two cookbooks that have been extremely helpful in cooking with my food allergies:

Bakin' Without Eggs by Rosemarie Emro

The Food Allergy News Cookbook: A Collection of Recipes from Food Allergy News and Members of the Food Allergy Network, edited by Anne Munoz-Furlong

Also, the members of the FARE Teen Advisory Group compiled a Teen Advisory Group Cookbook full of many of their favorite recipes (all of which are free of peanuts, tree nuts, fish and shellfish—and several are free of all eight major allergens).

IN CLOSING

This resource guide may not answer every question you have about food allergies. FARE and FAACT have Teen Advisory Groups (both of which I am a member of) that exist for the purpose of helping answer your questions and giving advice. There are also Facebook groups, monitored by teen advisors, for teens to post their comments, concerns, and experiences. These are places for teens to ask questions, give advice, find support, and make new friends.

And just to give you an idea of where the subject of food allergies stands today...

FOOD ALLERGIES IN 2013: A YEAR IN REVIEW

New auto-injectors became available. In 2013, two new epinephrine auto-injectors came on the market, providing more options to patients.

World Allergy Week and Food Safety Month were dedicated to food allergies. Demonstrating the growing prevalence and awareness that food allergies are a global public health issue, both World Allergy Week in May and Food Safety Month in September were dedicated to educating the public about food allergies.

Sports teams showed their support. Northwestern University hosted the first ever peanut-free college football game in 2013. Additionally, Major League Baseball teams across the country welcomed families managing food allergies for nut-free or nut-controlled games. The Seattle Mariners, along with other teams, even invited kids with food allergies to throw out the first pitch at games.

The Centers for Disease Control and Prevention (CDC) published the first national school food allergy guidelines. These guidelines are intended to support the implementation of school food allergy management policies in schools and early childhood programs and guide improvements to existing practices. Implementing these guidelines will help schools reduce allergic reactions, improve response to life-threatening situations and ensure current policies are in line with laws that protect children with serious health issues.

Celebrities raised awareness. Celebrities like Julie Bowen, Adrian Peterson, Jerome Bettis, Jo Frost and Kenton Duty stood up to help bring awareness to the serious nature of food allergies. They spoke up on talk shows and public service announcements, and told their stories about their connections to the cause. Additionally, prominent bloggers gathered for the first annual Food Allergy Bloggers Conference (FABlogCon) for a weekend of learning, support and inspiration.

FARE launched a public awareness campaign about food allergy bullying. During Food Allergy Awareness Week in May, FARE released a public service announcement about the growing concern of food allergy bullying. The video has more than 36,000 views on YouTube and has helped bring attention to the issue. In December, a bill was filed which would require schools to put in place a policy that addresses food allergy bullying.

The media shined the spotlight on food allergies. The New York Times made a splash with their "Allergy Busters" article about the latest treatment for food allergies. They also ran an opinion column by author Curtis Sittenfeld urging increased availability of epinephrine in schools. Anderson Cooper hosted teens Danielle and Lauren Mongeau, who advocated for the successful passage of a bill in Rhode Island that created a food allergy awareness training program for restaurants. Also related to restaurant awareness, FARE and the National Restaurant Association partnered to create the first comprehensive, interactive national training program for restaurant personnel to help them become more aware on the issue of food allergies.

The FARE Walk for Food Allergy had a record-breaking season. The 2013 FARE Walk for Food Allergy season was the largest in its history, raising $3.6 million for food allergy research, advocacy, awareness, and education—a $1.2 million dollar increase from 2012.

The Discovery Channel aired a special documentary about food allergy. Narrated by Steve Carell, this documentary explored what it's like to live with life-threatening food allergies, how families and individuals managing food allergies are working to raise awareness in their communities, and the vital research underway to find effective treatments and a cure.

The School Access to Emergency Epinephrine Act was signed into law. On November 13, President Obama signed this historic and potentially lifesaving legislation—the first federal law encouraging schools to stock epinephrine for use in allergic emergencies. At the signing ceremony, the president revealed that his own daughter, Malia, is allergic to peanuts.

My hope is that this resource guide will come in handy for those teenagers and pre-teens struggling through the trials and tribulations of food allergies. I want people to understand that while this condition is undeniably difficult to live with, having food allergies doesn't mean you can't have a normal life—even a good one. Because of this, I'm closing this book with a list (names you might recognize) of people who have fought the fight against food allergies and come out on the other side.

Zooey Deschanel: dairy, eggs and wheat
Serena Williams: peanuts
Billy Bob Thorton: shellfish
Kelis: peanuts
Ray Romano: peanuts
Joshua Jackson: peanuts and tree nuts
Halle Berry: shellfish
Alex Kapranos (Franz Ferdinand): peanuts
Clay Aiken: mint, shellfish, tree nuts, mushrooms and chocolate
Drew Barrymore: multiple food allergies (garlic and coffee)
Steve Martin: shellfish
Brianna Rhea Adkins (Trace Adkins' daughter): nuts, dairy and wheat
Mason Disick (Kourtney Kardashian's son): peanuts
Jayden Spears (Britney Spears' son): undisclosed
Jessica Simpson: cheese, tomato and wheat
Miley Cyrus: cinnamon
Kenton Duty: chocolate and wheat
Jo Frost: tree nuts, peanuts, crustaceans and rye
Adrian Peterson: shrimp, scallops and lobster
Oliver McLanahan Phillips (Julie Bowen's son): peanuts

BIBLIOGRAPHY

"Alerts and Ingredient Notices." Food Allergy Research and Education. Food Allergy Research and Education, n.d. Web. 2 July 2014.

"Anaphylaxis Emergency Action Plan." American Academy of Allergy, Asthma, and Immunology. American Academy of Allergy, Asthma, and Immunology, July 2013. Web. 30 June 2014.

"Bus Drivers and Transportation Checklist." Food Allergy and Anaphylaxis Connection Team. Legend Web Works, Dec. 2013. Web. 30 June 2014.

California Innovations. N.p., n.d. Web. 29 July 2014.

Centers for Disease Control and Prevention. Voluntary Guidelines for Managing Food Allergies in Schools and Early Care and Education Programs. Washington, DC: US Department of Health and Human Services; 2013.

Coleman. Coleman Company, n.d. Web. 8 July 2014.

"College and University Food Services." Food Allergy and Anaphylaxis Connection Team. Legend Web Works, n.d. Web. 2 July 2014.

"College and University Guidelines for Managing Students with Food Allergies." Food Allergy Research and Education. Food Allergy Research and Education, n.d. Web. 2 July 2014.

"EpiPen4Schools." Bioridge Pharma. Mylan Specialty, n.d. Web. 30 June 2014.

"Facts and Statistics." Food Allergy Research and Education. Food Allergy Research and Education, n.d. Web. 2 July 2014.

"FARE College Food Allergy Program." Food Allergy Research and Education. Food Allergy Research and Education, n.d. Web. 2 July 2014.

"FARE College Summits." Food Allergy Research and Education. Food Allergy Research and Education, n.d. Web. 2 July 2014.
"Field Trips." Food Allergy and Anaphylaxis Connection Team. Legend Web Works, n.d. Web. 2 July 2014.

Fitterman, Lisa. "Dating with Allergies, a Tricky Business." Allergic Living. AGW Publishing, n.d. Web. 2 July 2014.

"Food Allergen Labeling and Consumer Protection Act." Food Allergy and Anaphylaxis Connection Team. Legend Web Works, n.d. Web. 2 July 2014.

"Food Allergies in 2013: A Year in Review." FARE Blog. N.p., 2 Jan. 2014. Web. 10 July 2014.

"Food Allergy and Anaphylaxis Emergency Care Plan." Food Allergy Research & Education. Food Allergy Research & Education, n.d. Web. 2 July 2014.

"Food Allergy Management and Education." St. Louis Children's Hospital. Washington University School of Medicine, n.d. Web. 30 June 2014. (FAACT references FAME, a program created by the St. Louis Children's Hospital)

"Food Labels." Food Allergy and Anaphylaxis Connection Team. Legend Web Works, n.d. Web. 2 July 2014.

"For School Personnel." Food Allergy and Anaphylaxis Connection Team. Legend Web Works, n.d. Web. 2 July 2014.

Goldberg, Stacy. "Do's and Don'ts of Dating Someone with a Food Allergy." Fox News 11 Feb. 2013: n. pag. Fox News Magazine. Web. 2 July 2014.

"Government Relations National and Statewide School Guidelines." Food Allergy and Anaphylaxis Connection Team. Legend Web Works, n.d. Web. 2 July 2014.

"Guidelines for Managing Food Allergies at Camp." Food Allergy Research and Education. Food Allergy Research and Education, n.d. Web. 2 July 2014.

Igloo. Igloo Products, n.d. Web. 8 July 2014.

Keep Cool Bags. Keep Cool Bags, n.d. Web. 29 July 2014.

Koko Lunch Bags. Kokolunchbags.org, n.d. Web. 8 July 2014.

Koolatron. Koolatron, n.d. Web. 8 July 2014.

Lands' End. Lands' End, n.d. Web. 2 July 2014.

MedicAlert Foundation. MedicAlert Foundation, n.d. Web. 10 July 2014.

MedicAlert Foundation. MedicAlert Foundation, n.d. Web. 10 July 2014.

Paz, Krisha. "Kiss Me If You Can: Food Allergies and the First Date." College and Cook 1 Feb. 2014: n. pag. College and Cook. Web. 30 July 2014.

"Resources for College Students." Food Allergy Research and Education. Food Allergy Research and Education, n.d. Web. 2 July 2014.

"Resources for Teens." Food Allergy Research and Education. Food Allergy Research and Education, n.d. Web. 2 July 2014.

"Restaurants." Food Allergy and Anaphylaxis Connection Team. Legend Web Works, n.d. Web. 2 July 2014.

SafeFARE. Food Allergy Research & Education, n.d. Web. 28 July 2014.

"SafeFARE: Chef Card Template." Food Allergy Research and Education. Food Allergy Research and Education, n.d. Web. 2 July 2014.

"Scott H. Sicherer." Mount Sinai Hospital. Icahn School of Medicine at Mount Sinai, n.d. Web. 23 July 2014.

"Section 504 Plans." Food Allergy and Anaphylaxis Connection Team. Legend Web Works, n.d. Web. 30 June 2014.

"Statewide Restaurant Legislation." Food Allergy and Anaphylaxis Connection Team. Legend Web Works, n.d. Web. 2 July 2014.

"Teacher's Checklist for Managing Food Allergies." Food Allergy Research and Education. Food Allergy Research and Education, n.d. Web. 2 July 2014.

"28 Celebrities with Allergies." Allermates & Medimates. Awearables, 7 May 2012. Web. 10 July 2014.

United States Department of Justice Civil Rights Division. Introduction to the ADA. Washington: GPO. Information and Technical Assistance on the Americans with Disabilities Act. Web. 30 June 2014. (referred to by the FAACT website)

U.S. Department of Health and Human Services. Food Allergen Labeling And Consumer Protection Act of 2004 Questions and Answers. Washington: GPO. U.S. Food and Drug Administration. Web. 30 June 2014.

ADDITIONAL SOURCES FOR MORE INFORMATION

Centers for Disease Control and Prevention. Voluntary Guidelines for Managing Food Allergies in Schools and Early

Care and Education Programs Frequently Asked Questions. Washington, DC: US Department of Health and Human Services; 2013.

"Food Services." Food Allergy and Anaphylaxis Connection Team. Legend Web Works, n.d. Web. 2 July 2014.

"Government Relations School Access to Emergency Epinephrine Federal Legislation." Food Allergy and Anaphylaxis Connection Team. Legend Web Works, n.d. Web. 2 July 2014.

Living Confidently with Food Allergy Handbook. N.p.: Anaphylaxis Canada, n.d. Newly Diagnosed Support Centre Anaphylaxis Canada. Web. 2 July 2014.

"Managing Food Allergies in the School Setting." Food Allergy Research and Education. Food Allergy Research and Education, n.d. Web. 2 July 2014.

Public Law 108–282—AUG. 2, 2004. Washington: GPO. U.S. Food and Drug Administration. Web. 30 June 2014. (referenced by FAACT)
"Teens and Kids with Food Allergies Need to be Careful About Kissing." Kids with Food Allergies. Kids with Food Allergies, July 2008. Web. 2 July 2014.

United States. United States Department of Agriculture Food and Nutrition Service. Accommodating Children with Special Dietary Needs in the School Nutrition Programs Guidance for School Food Service Staff. Washington: GPO, n.d. Print.

U.S. Department of Health and Human Services National Institutes of Health. Guidelines for the Diagnosis and Management of Food Allergy in the United States. Doc. 11-7699. National Institute of Allergy and Infectious Diseases, 2011. National Institute of Allergy and Infectious Diseases. Web. 2 July 2014.